The BIG "Lit-tle Gua Sha Book

Learning (and Loving) the Ancient Healing Art of *Gua Sha*

by

Leta Herman
& Jaye McElroy

Authors of
THE ENERGY OF LOVE
and CONNECTING YOUR CIRCLE

For online videos, tutorials, and classes, visit:
www.GuaShaBook.com

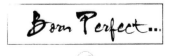

Northampton, Massachusetts

Important: The information and techniques discussed in this book are based upon the personal and professional experiences and research of its authors. The information contained in this book is not meant to be a substitute for medical care by a physician or other health care provider(s). Any diagnosis or medical care should be done under the guidance of a health care professional. The publisher does not promote the use of specific health care protocols but believes the information in this book should be made available to the general public. Neither the authors nor the publisher assume any liability whatsoever for the use of the information (or inability to use the information) contained in this book. The authors and publisher strongly suggest consulting a physician or professional health care provider about the appropriateness of any technique or procedure mentioned in this book.

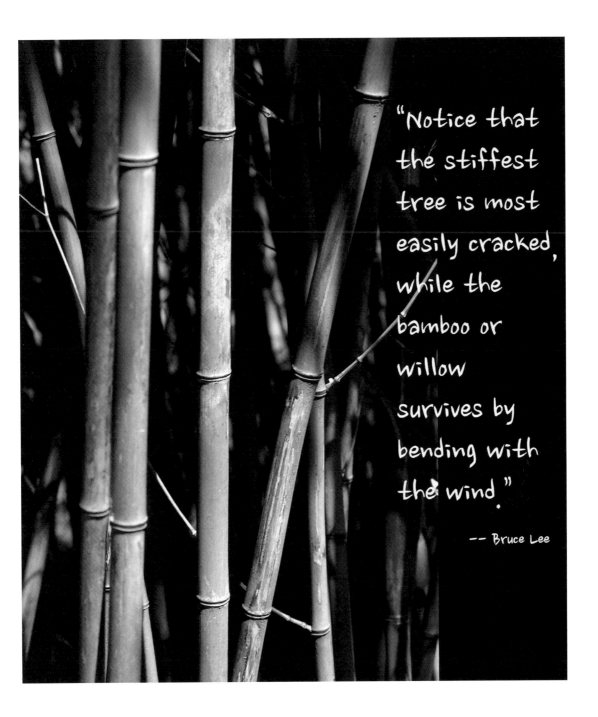

"Notice that the stiffest tree is most easily cracked, while the bamboo or willow survives by bending with the wind."

-- Bruce Lee

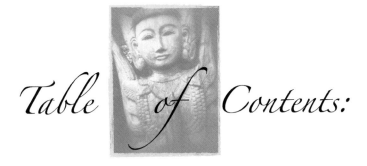

Table of Contents:

WHY WE WROTE THIS BOOK

The ancient healing art of *Gua Sha* has always been fascinating to me as a Chinese Medicine practitioner. I love teaching it and sharing the knowledge. I added the *Gua Sha* technique to my acupressure practice over 10 years ago after studying with Jeffrey Yuen, an inspiring and amazing Chinese Medicine teacher and 88th-generation Daoist priest. Over the past 10 years, my understanding of *Gua Sha* has continued to grow, and I keep an open mind and learn new things every day.

Recently, I asked my writing partner Jaye McElroy, who has become quite a skilled *Gua Sha*-er herself, to join me in teaching *Gua Sha* workshops. We both enjoyed compiling the material so much (and found so little written on the topic) that we decided to put it all together into this "BIG" book in a "Little" package that anyone could benefit from reading. (That's why we decided to call it *The BIG "Little" Book of Gua Sha*.)

Our goal for this book is to give readers all they need to get started with *Gua Sha*. *Gua Sha* is really easy and provides astounding benefits with such little effort. It is so advantageous, I can't believe more people don't already know about it in the West. Hopefully this book will change that fact and get more people interested. Jaye and I both hope you will find *Gua Sha* just as amazing as we have. Grab a spoon and let's go!

Happy spooning!

HOW TO USE
THIS BOOK

This book is made up of Five Chapters, a Conclusion, and a Glossary.

Chapter 1 describes *Gua Sha* and its history.

Chapter 2 provides an introduction to energy (*Qi*) and explains how tension and resistance get stuck in your body.

Chapter 3 covers all you need to know before you begin.

Chapter 4 walks you through how to perform *Gua Sha*.

Chapter 5 goes over advanced techniques for working with specific ailments and pain.

We end with a Conclusion and a Glossary of key terms that you can refer to while reading the book.

If you are new to Chinese Medicine, you may find some of the more advanced material a little difficult. We highly recommend that enthusiasts purchase a book about the Chinese Medicine meridians of the body or do some research online to better understand the primary meridian system. While you do not need to learn all 365 acu-points on the body to do *Gua Sha*, knowing a bit about some of the meridians will help you become more skilled at using *Gua Sha* to help yourself and your loved ones. We hope the many photos and illustrations in this step-by-step book will make *Gua Sha* easy for you to do! To view video examples of *Gua Sha* or to take an on-line class, please go to: www.GuaShaBook.com.

YOU WANT TO DO WHAT WITH THAT SPOON?

Some practitioners call it *scraping*. Some call it *frictioning* or *coining*. Others call it *spooning*. We're not talking about snuggling with your sweetie in bed. We're talking about an ancient folk medicine technique that the Chinese call *Gua Sha* (both *Gua* and *Sha* rhyme with "draw").

In Chinese, *Gua* means to scrape or rub and *Sha* represents the toxic energy that is released when the technique causes blood to flush to the surface of the skin, thus making red splotchy marks that typically last several days on the body. Some Chinese call it *Gua Feng*, or "scrape wind," which is a more literal translation because the technique releases the type of energy that the Chinese call "wind" or "*feng*." We will talk more about *Wind* in the body later in the book. First let's take a brief look at the history of this ancient healing art form.

History of *Gua Sha*

Gua Sha has been used for thousands of years to heal many different types of ailments. It may have originated in the area that used to be

Southern China but is modern-day Vietnam. Families learned to master *Gua Sha* as a useful and powerful way to heal themselves, their families, and friends. For more serious illnesses or injuries that required a doctor, *Gua Sha* was useful in villages for relieving symptoms until a traveling physician came to town. The earliest recorded *Gua Sha* tools appear to have been rhinoceros horns. Later, people used buffalo and oxen horns. These horns have inherent cooling properties built into them, which help draw heat and toxins out of the skin.

There are literally hundreds of different *Gua Sha* tools (the image opposite shows some of the more common tools). Today, they are made of various stone materials, stainless steel, and even titanium. In Hong Kong, I visited a booth at an outdoor market where all the merchants' tables were completely covered with every conceivable variety of *Gua Sha* tool you could imagine and then some! I saw tools made from buffalo horn, goat horn, jade, dark stone, metal, and even plastic. Tools are also made for different parts of the body (long flat sticks with notches in them, for example, especially made for boney fingers and delicate toes). There were also some very strange shapes there! Rounded tools, comb-shaped tools made out of jade, heart-shaped tools, tools shaped like a crown, horns that were carved into different horn-like shapes, and many other amorphous shapes in big and small sizes.

As a practitioner of *Gua Sha*, I have tried many, many *Gua Sha* tools over the years. I suggest beginners experiment and try out some different tools. See what works best for you, your hand, and your clients. For me, I have found a porcelain soupspoon works amazingly well.

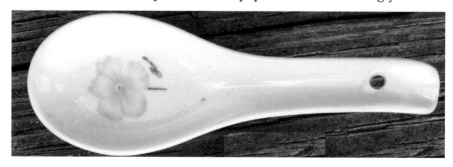

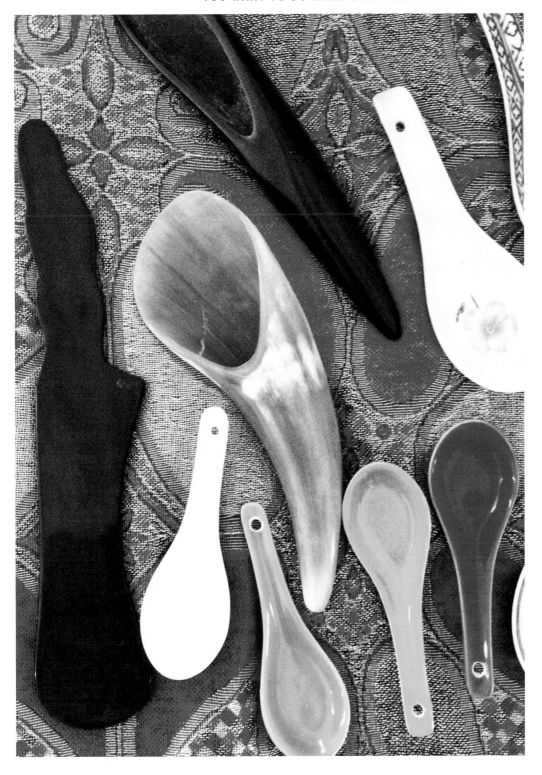

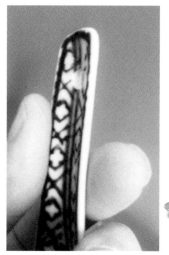

These spoons are easily found in Asian grocery stores worldwide. The rounded edges and the ergonomic design keep my hand from cramping and allow me to maneuver my wrist around different bony areas on the body. You can even turn it around and use the handle for small crevices like the area next to the collarbone.

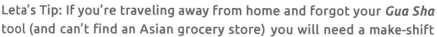

Leta's Tip: Be careful not to cause pain when using the smaller end of the spoon. It's more pointed, so requires much less pressure.

Leta's Tip: If you're traveling away from home and forgot your *Gua Sha* tool (and can't find an Asian grocery store) you will need a make-shift tool. Go to the kitchen or local grocery store and look at all the jars you can find. It's the lids you need to look at! Search for a lid that has a smooth edge (not ridged like the plastic lids used for most peanut butter jars). Smooth metal lids used for baby food or jelly jars can work in a jam (pun intended!). Also, I have used olive oil from the kitchen when I did not have coconut oil handy. It works well and might even make you crave Italian food for dinner!

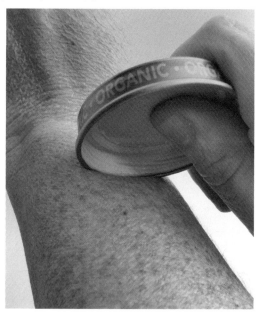

What does *Gua Sha* do to the body?

With the proper technique and an appropriate tool, the actual motion of scraping the skin *releases* the surface of the skin to promote circulation of blood and energy called *Qi*, pronounced "chee". Oddly, it can make the skin look like you're covered with bizarre hickies or a big, red rash. I still haven't come up with a more descriptive word that's better than "hickey!" In fact, when I do a small amount of *Gua Sha* on someone's neck, I often jokingly warn them that they're going to have some explaining to do at home.

Gua Sha might **look** like it hurts but it's completely painless in 95% of the cases. On occasion, some people find it temporarily uncomfortable or even ticklish, but if they stick with it, the odd feeling usually stops. Many people love the feeling of having *Gua Sha* done and say it feels like a really good massage.

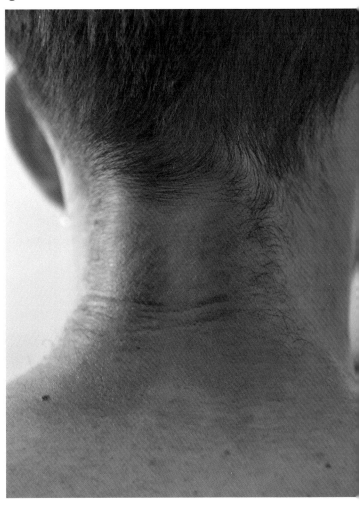

Leta's Tip: Always start with a light touch and gradually increase the pressure, even with people who are used to having the treatments. Let the person's sensitivity on each specific day guide your spooning.

What exactly *are* those dark red marks?

Practitioners and healers often call the redness that emerges when the skin is scraped the "*Sha*." In Western Medicine, the technical term for this hickey-like redness is called *Petechiae*, which means tiny red spots containing blood just under the surface of the skin. The redness is actually the blood rising to the surface as energy is released.

The petechiae–redness–or "*Sha*" as many people like to call it, is a sign that toxic Wind energy is present below the surface of the skin and is now being released. I always say to clients, "Yay! You have giant red marks on your back! Don't be alarmed. That's good news!" The red marks will **ONLY** appear if you have stuck energy. I am always amazed that I can spoon/scrape one area for a very long time and no petechiae or *Sha* appears at all. Yet, on another part of the same person's body, I can do *Gua Sha* and get a huge amount of redness in a very short time.

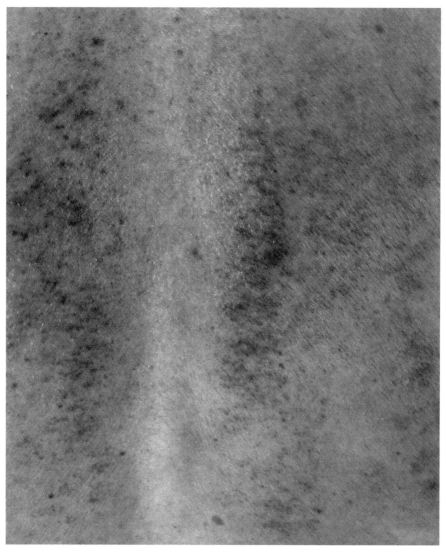

Leta's Tip: Many *Gua Sha* beginners see the skin turn slightly red with no visible red dots (petechiae) and stop, thinking that is the *Sha*. The redness they're seeing is not *Sha*. It's redness that a light massage would bring out. You have to see actual red spots emerge.

What is *Gua Sha* actually good for?

Wow, that is such a big question! In this book, we are just going to cover some basics. Think of this book as *Gua Sha* 101. It will cover the things you need to learn to start on the path of becoming a more advanced healer. We will explain in more detail some of the more advanced uses for *Gua Sha* later in this book, but here is just a short list of more common conditions *Gua Sha* can help with:

Colds – Preventing colds before they even start

Flu – Helping move flu out of the body faster

Fevers – Reducing high fevers

Pulled Muscles – Healing aching muscles, muscle/tendon strains, pinched nerves

Neck Pain – Healing all sorts of neck pain

Shoulder Pain – Healing shoulder and scapula pain

Back Pain – Healing all sorts of back pain (upper, mid, and lower)

Repetitive Stress – Healing repetitive stress pain in the limbs

Carpal Tunnel – Healing carpal tunnel pain or other nerve entrapments

Numbness and Tingling – Healing numbness and tingling in the fingers

Shin Splints – Removing shin splints

Plantar Fasciitis – Healing plantar fasciitis

Cough – Relieving severe cough

Migraines – Relieving migraines and headaches

Stress – Releasing areas of stress and tense/tight muscles

Injuries – Faster recovery from injuries

Aging – Promoting circulation in the skin, making it more youthful

Shingles – Relieving symptoms from shingles

Poison Ivy – Relieving itchiness from poison ivy

Allergies – Relieving itchy eyes, runny nose, and scratchy throat

As you can see, *Gua Sha* is a pretty handy technique for families with children to have on hand to help alleviate poison ivy, frequent colds, and many small injuries. *Gua Sha* is very popular today across Asia, especially in China, Taiwan, and Vietnam, as well as in Indonesia, Cambodia, Laos, and Thailand, where families often perform it on each other regularly.

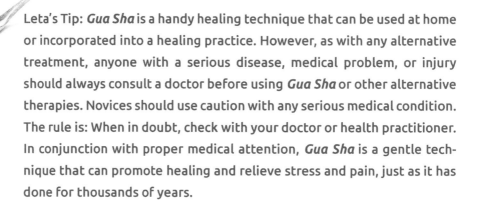 Leta's Tip: *Gua Sha* is a handy healing technique that can be used at home or incorporated into a healing practice. However, as with any alternative treatment, anyone with a serious disease, medical problem, or injury should always consult a doctor before using *Gua Sha* or other alternative therapies. Novices should use caution with any serious medical condition. The rule is: When in doubt, check with your doctor or health practitioner. In conjunction with proper medical attention, *Gua Sha* is a gentle technique that can promote healing and relieve stress and pain, just as it has done for thousands of years.

Chapter

2

SAY *CHEE-SE*, PLEASE

To explain this big idea of Qi (or *chi*, pronounced like "chee" in cheese), we're going to have to cover a little science first. There are some people who spend their entire lives studying this "stuff," so think of this as a quick primer for all the most important answers of life. Hah! If only it were that simple!

What is *qi* ?

Thousands of years ago (exactly how long no one really knows but probably 3000 years), ancient Chinese philosophers developed theories about *qi*. Similar to how our modern physicists observe nature to develop theories of velocity and relativity, these philosophers examined the synchronicity of life and the delicate balance of living creatures on the planet. They believed the most important thing that every living being on the planet shared was . . . ENERGY. Let's try to understand energy and the lessons that the ancient teachers tried to impart.

Go with the *flow* . . .

Energy moves in humans like the electricity delivered to power outlets in our houses. You can't actually *see* the electricity. You can't grasp it, although it can electrocute you if you get too close. You can't smell it—well, if you do, it's time to call the Fire Department! But, seriously, you know it's there because it turns on lamps, heats toasters, and makes all our TVs and computers work like magic. But short of sticking your finger in the socket to actually *feel* electricity's power, we all believe it's there even if we can't see it.

In all living organisms, including you, *qi* is the energy coursing within you. It's your electricity, so to speak. It flows through you and radiates from you. All humans have their own set of internal power lines, and if you put a person's power lines all together, they form a

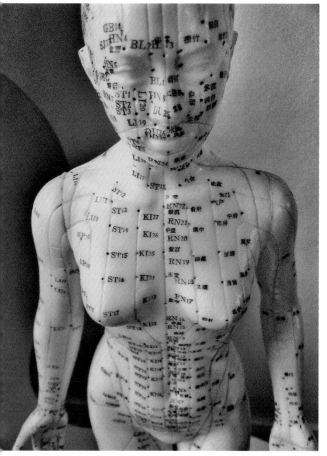

power grid in the body. These power grids, in humans, are called *meridians*.

Covering your body, meridians have points (kind of like electrical outlets) that allow you to plug into or access and stimulate your energy. These points are called *acu-points*. They are the points that Chinese Medicine practitioners use (in acupressure or acupuncture) for energy healing work and treatments.

Your *qi* is your power and your life source, animating your body. It's the reason you move the way you do. Ancient Chinese masters created a vocabulary to describe the movement of *qi*. The most basic movements of *qi* are Yin and Yang.

The *Taijitu yin/yang* symbol can be seen throughout the world, from ancient monasteries to the bottoms of kids' skateboards. But many people don't know what the symbol actually means or signifies. Do you know? (Wait! You don't have to run off to Google it . . . we will tell you!)

This famous *yin/yang* symbol shows you the simplest movements of energy flowing upward and outward (*yang* energy) as well as downward and inward (*yin* energy). Think of how heat always rises. As heat rises, cooler air descends. This is how *yin* (cooler, denser) and *yang* (hotter, expansive) energy flows in life.

When Wind blows! (Literally and figuratively)

Wind is a metaphor for the kind of *energy* we're trying to release when doing *Gua Sha*. The best translation of Wind (*feng*) is resistance or tension. Imagine standing on a mountaintop where a cold wind is blowing fiercely. You will instinctively have an impulse to brace against the wind by tensing up and shrugging your shoulders up to your neck. It's a natural reaction to ward off the wind—our bodies know that we can "catch a cold" when there are temperature changes carried by a strong wind. Our reaction is a learned response.

This reaction creates tension that you put into your muscles. This tension doesn't always release right away as it should. When you get home, you might suddenly have a pain in your neck (literally) from the tension you just created when trying to stave off the cold wind! This tension is what the Chinese call Wind. The idea is that the blowing wind got stuck in you when you braced against it. But truly, it's you that got stuck as you were trying to ward off the mighty wind.

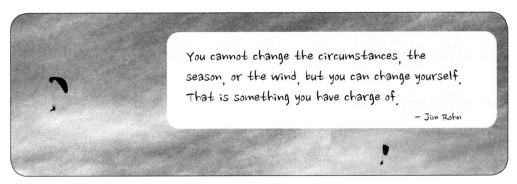

You cannot change the circumstances, the season, or the wind, but you can change yourself. That is something you have charge of.

— Jim Rohn

To explain it even further, it means that your *qi* and blood became stagnant in your shoulders when the muscles engaged in isometric tightness. Afterwards, energy was blocked and no longer flowing in that tight, tense area, and voilà—you have a sore neck.

Whenever our bodies react to germs (or climatic conditions that bring on a cold), we automatically and unconsciously resist these invaders. We get Wind because we're starting to feel sick, and our bodies are trying to fight the sickness. We feel tension in the back of our necks, our throats start to get sore as they tighten, and our eyes itch. These are all signs of Wind penetrating and being stirred up in our bodies.

The most common use of *Gua Sha* is to release the Wind *before* the cold starts. Wind is resistance to a cold that gets trapped in your body, and it needs to get out! Amazingly, if you *Gua Sha* the back of your neck, the tops of your shoulders, and between your shoulder blades, you may often prevent a cold before it even starts.

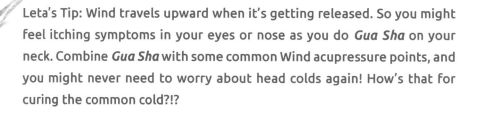

Leta's Tip: Wind travels upward when it's getting released. So you might feel itching symptoms in your eyes or nose as you do *Gua Sha* on your neck. Combine *Gua Sha* with some common Wind acupressure points, and you might never need to worry about head colds again! How's that for curing the common cold?!?

Wind is also prevalent when you injure yourself or overdo activities that involve heavy muscle, tendon, and ligament activity. The tension comes with injuries because you're trying to avoid pain. You anticipate the pain and even brace and wince before you actually experience the expected pain. This resistance and tension cause more pain than the actual injury! One of the secrets I've learned from years of learning and practicing *Kung Fu* is that when you are injured, you need to minimize your own Wind response (relaxing instead of bracing, wincing, or contracting your muscles). If you relax after an injury, you will recover not just one or two days earlier than usual, but in just a fraction of the time.

Resistance is a self-defeating reaction. For example, injuries that usually take a week or more to heal might take only a day or two without resistance.

To ice or not to ice: That is the question!

One of the places where Western and Eastern medicine really don't agree is on the use of ice. While ice can calm down the resistance (by reducing the pain initially after the accident and stopping contraction), it also reduces *qi* flow and drives any Wind that is present **deeper** into the area, making the injury take much longer to heal. Think about it from a more scientific point of view . . . cold slows down molecules in any situation. Apply cold to your body, and you're slowing down *qi* flow. Slowed *qi* flow usually creates stagnation and eventually pain and illness.

Instead of using ice on an injury, the ancient Chinese created a cold liniment that smells like menthol called *Zheng Gu Shui* (pronounced Jung Goo Shway) with many Chinese herbs that soothe the inflammation *while* releasing the Wind. *Zheng Gu Shui* literally means "Water that Fixes Your Bones." It encourages the flow of *qi* instead of slowing it down the way applying ice does. It is common practice for healers to create their own recipe, each slightly different but still very similar. After the injury has improved, (and it's safe to do *Gua Sha*), the *Gua Sha* usually takes care of the last bit of pain that might remain in the affected area.

Six degrees of pain

Mostly, *Gua Sha* is a pleasant experience. Mostly. We say that with some hesitation. Everyone and every body is different. *Gua Sha* can feel like a soothing massage to some and somewhat painful to others. The technique is not about bruising the area or digging deeply into the skin! The correct technique uses a scooping and lifting action at a 30 to 45 degree angle. The technique relies on lifting energy out of the muscles through the skin. Think of it like a loofah, scraping off a top layer verses penetrating into the muscles.

Occasionally, a person may find the treatment uncomfortable. Be attentive to the recipient's responses and needs, lightening the pressure when the person is uncomfortable and proceeding delicately and cautiously. You might need a session or two before the recipient can allow you to use full pressure.

Leta's Tip: Don't try to rush the cure. The redness (petechiae) has to disappear or dissipate completely before the next *Gua Sha* session.

A small percentage of people find *Gua Sha* quite painful. Typically, these people would also find any kind of massage or rubbing painful. But if they continue with treatments, usually the pain subsides once the *Sha* (redness) appears. However, some people cannot tolerate *Gua Sha* and refuse the treatment due to their discomfort from it. I always respect that. Perhaps the old saying, "Different strokes for different folks" applies here.

Some people find *Gua Sha* quite ticklish. This ticklishness can be an indicator of where the *Sha* or "Wind" is located in their body. In other words, this is exactly where they need to have *Gua Sha* performed! Once the scraping is done, the area is usually no longer ticklish.

Chapter 3

ZONING IN ON THE ZONES

It is important to explain to a new recipient what *Gua Sha* will look and feel like before an initial session.

Seeing RED is a very good thing!

Make sure the recipient understands that there will be red markings—sometimes a lot of red marks—that may last for 2 to 4 days. (In some rare cases they can last up to a week.) Explain that it's not bruising due to pressure (although bruising may result if you use too much pressure), but that you will use light pressure with a technique that brings blood to the surface as energy is released. Ask whether the recipient is ready to proceed with the treatment and tell them they have the power to stop if it's uncomfortable.

Once a young woman informed me just before I was going to start a *Gua Sha* session on her back that she was going to her prom that night with an open-back dress! Needless to say, we made an appointment for another day. She was grateful at the end of her next session that we hadn't done it the first day because her entire back was red, red, red! Teachers, business people, and performers may be particularly concerned about the red marks on their necks and arms, so I always make sure it's okay for *Gua Sha* to be performed before starting a session. Most people are interested, sometimes even happy, with their markings. I often offer to take a picture of their backs with their smartphones so they can see the results right away.

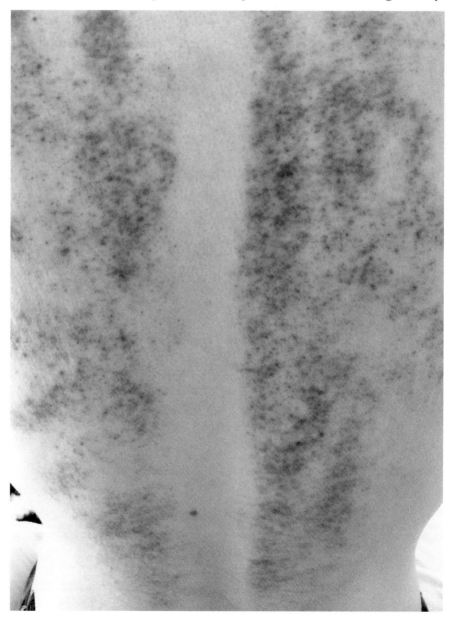

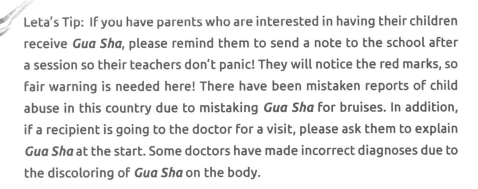

Leta's Tip: If you have parents who are interested in having their children receive *Gua Sha*, please remind them to send a note to the school after a session so their teachers don't panic! They will notice the red marks, so fair warning is needed here! There have been mistaken reports of child abuse in this country due to mistaking *Gua Sha* for bruises. In addition, if a recipient is going to the doctor for a visit, please ask them to explain *Gua Sha* at the start. Some doctors have made incorrect diagnoses due to the discoloring of *Gua Sha* on the body.

Staying in the red zone

Whenever someone is coming down with a cold, has a cold, or is experiencing muscle pain, consider doing *Gua Sha*, either on the actual location of the pain or in three main *zones* where *Gua Sha* is commonly used to release Wind.

- **Zone 1** – Back of neck, good for when you're just getting a cold

- **Zone 2** – Between the shoulder blades, good for more serious colds or pain in the back

- **Zone 3** – Under the breasts and around the sides of the ribs, good for flus or viruses

In addition to these zones, you can look at areas of the body that might have signs that *Gua Sha* would be useful. Look for areas of the body, especially on the back, that are tight and raised (like a large raised area). These are areas where the muscles are particularly tense and stuck.

You can also examine the skin itself. Often you may see a hint of something that looks like petechiae (red dots) in an area. You can also press your fingers on the skin and let go. Wherever the white marks disappear more slowly is likely an area that may need some *Gua Sha* work.

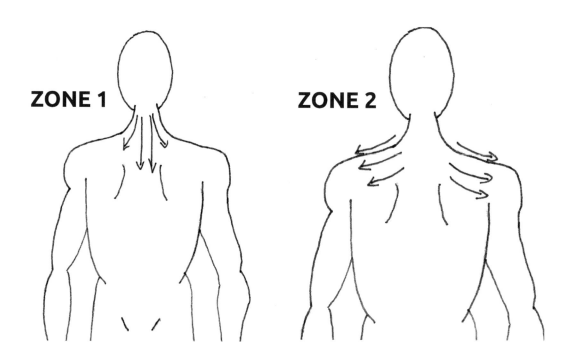

ZONE 1

ZONE 2

Leta's Tip: If you're not sure where to start, no worries. Just try doing *Gua Sha* in one area, and it will tell you soon enough whether you're on the right track. Redness? Keep it up a little longer (about 30 to 60 seconds is usually enough or until no more redness is emerging). No redness? Move to another location on the body. Whatever area starts to show the *Sha*, follow it to the edges and continue until you get to an area with no red. In other words, keep it in the red zone!

Different strokes for different folks!

The *Gua Sha* technique I use (and teach) has three levels of pressure:

1. Light - Use very light pressure to release the energy. This technique is used most often with children and the elderly. You should also use this pressure with anyone who is very ill or weak. With light pressure, you're not trying to get a lot of Sha (redness) out. You're simply trying to release a small amount of energy. Start with light, small, and quick strokes simply to stimulate the skin, energy, and blood in the area. If the person does well with very light pressure, you can increase the pressure slightly until a small amount of Sha comes out. Make sure the person is not experiencing any discomfort.

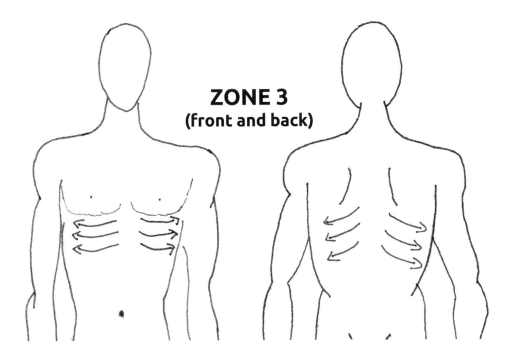

ZONE 3
(front and back)

2. **Medium** - Most *Gua Sha* is done with medium pressure. It's still fairly light, and really focuses on a scooping action to release the *Sha*. With medium pressure, the person should have little or no visible bruises the next day, only redness.

3. **Heavy** - Occasionally a person who is very strong (it's like their energy is fit to burst) has tons and tons of *Sha* all over their body. You can use more pressure, and the *Sha* will turn purple. But heavy pressure is still not intended to bruise. It's just shy of bruising. *Gua Sha* should never hurt due to the pressure that you are using. It's an energy treatment, not a pressure treatment.

Say yes! to the safe word…"Stop!"

In the beginning of any session, especially with a new recipient, you should agree upon a safe word practice. "Stop!" is the word of choice since it is universally understood. Grunts, groans, wiggling, and even swearing are common. But make sure they know that if they need to actually stop due to the level of discomfort or pain, they can use the "safe" word and feel comfortable knowing you will respect it. Many people will relax when they know they are in control and can suspend an activity if they feel the need to. It's also important to ask them frequently during the session how the treatment feels to make sure you're correctly attuned to their comfort level.

Journey to the center of the pain

We often do *Gua Sha* on the fleshier parts of the body or over wide, flat bony areas, such as the shoulder blades. The *Sha* will often rise up more easily over bony areas than the deep fleshy areas. You will need more pressure on the fleshier areas, especially the buttocks and hips.

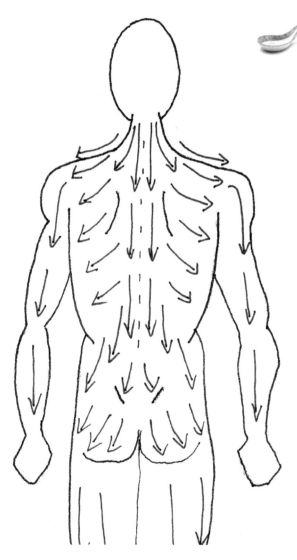

Leta's Tip: My general rule when doing **Gua Sha** is that you should work away from the center of the body. Also, if you plan to work on both the back and the front, start on the back and finish working on the front.

GUA SHA DIRECTIONS (back of the body)

The direction of *Gua Sha* strokes on the back is down the back of the neck, across the top of the shoulders towards the arms, down the back (avoiding the spine itself), outwards toward the sides of the ribs, down the buttocks, outwards toward the hips, down the back of the legs (avoiding the back of the knees), down to the ankles, and even down the backs of the feet.

GUA SHA DIRECTIONS
(front of the body)

The direction of *Gua Sha* on the front of the body is down the front of the neck (very lightly . . . it's a sensitive area due to bones and glands), lightly scrape out the collar bone towards the arms (toxins can often pool in that area), down the chest (good for cough, numbness, tingling, or muscle strains in the thumb or middle finger but otherwise it is not an area that should be *Gua Sha*'d much), under the breast area over the front of the ribs (good for flu-like symptoms), over the hip and psoas muscles if there is front leg strain, down the thighs and along the tibia (especially for shin splints), and down lightly into the foot.

Due to the redness that appears on the surface of the skin when the *Sha* is released, I do not generally apply *Gua Sha* to the face. However, there are many who believe *Gua Sha* can increase youthfulness in the face and neck and release tension in the skin that causes wrinkles and aging.

Mostly *Gua Sha* is performed downward and outward (away from the center). The exceptions to this rule include:

• **At the occiput** (the very bottom of the skull on the back of the neck)—the treatment sometimes works better if you go upward into the back of the skull from the neck over the muscles that attach there.
(see next page)

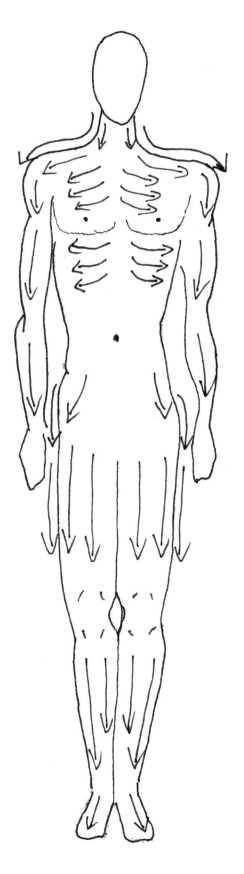

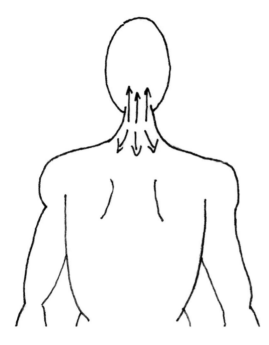

GUA SHA DIRECTIONS
(back of neck)

You can even do *Gua Sha* on the scalp right over the hair all around the head. Some *Gua Sha* tools look like a comb specifically for applying the technique to the scalp. Since you cannot see whether any redness is coming out, you should do *Gua Sha* on the scalp for 15–20 seconds over each area.

• **Around rashes**—such as poison ivy or shingles. In this case you're moving the energy away from the rash, circularly outward.

• **With injuries**—When there is swelling or bruising, the proper flow of energy can sometimes be restored by moving the energy away from the injury (circularly outward). It also helps to direct the *Gua Sha* along the flow of the energy meridian lines. Some meridians flow upward, and others flow downward. It can be a good idea to move the energy upward above an injured area if the direction of the channel is also moving upward in that area. For example, an injury on the inner ankle may need some upward *Gua Sha* because the Liver, Spleen, and Kidney meridians all travel up the leg from the inner ankle.

The spoon does not lie!

In Chinese Medicine, one of the most important concepts is that the cause of pain is not always where you actually feel the pain. The problem can be much more complex than what it appears to be on the surface. Different instances of pain can be better helped by understanding the Chinese meridians of energy and how energy flows through them in the body.

A good practice is to treat the affected meridian as well as the pain area itself. For example, if you have wrist pain, determine what meridian is closest to the painful area and follow that meridian further up the arm with your *Gua Sha* technique to see if redness emerges there. The pain in the wrist may result from a blockage of *qi* higher up above the wrist and the *Sha* will emerge in the area that's the true source of the pain. I often see the cause of a pain is some distance away, and the person is surprised.

No, no way, uh-uh . . . just don't

In our research of the history of *Gua Sha*, we read over and over that *Gua Sha* has never **caused** any injury to a person in its long history. However, we feel it's wise to be cautious in a number of cases. There are a number of contraindications to consider before you utilize your new skills.

Do NOT *Gua Sha* in the following cases

• **On pregnant women (unless you are a certified acupressurist or licensed acupuncturist – and then *only* in safe areas of the body).** If a woman is pregnant, it's important not to do *Gua Sha* anywhere on the belly. A practitioner may do a small amount of *Gua Sha* for muscle strains in the upper back, arms, or hips. There are many points of the body that can induce labor, so extreme care must be taken. This is also true for anyone doing massage or energywork with pregnant women.

• **On someone with blood disorders (such as inability to clot or excessive bruising).** Because *Gua Sha* causes blood to rise to the surface, do not perform it on people who have illnesses that impact the blood. Ask if the person has a blood disorder. Also ask whether the person has any trouble clotting or bruises easily or excessively. As a general rule, do not perform *Gua Sha* on someone who has any of the above issues. You may refer the person to a professional Chinese Medicine practitioner for *Gua Sha*.

• **On someone taking blood thinners.** Blood thinners may cause too much blood to rise to the surface when performing *Gua Sha*.

• **On someone with a communicable disease.** To ensure you do not contract a communicable disease, do not perform *Gua Sha* on a person who has a communicable disease. You may refer the person to a professional Chinese Medicine practitioner if *Gua Sha* is requested.

- **On someone with phlebitis (inflammation of a vein) or deep vein thrombosis.** Even if the person doesn't have phlebitis or thrombosis (conditions that involve swollen veins), it's a good idea to not perform *Gua Sha* over veins that are visibly swollen or purple.

Do NOT *Gua Sha* in the following areas

- **Over recent injuries or surgery.** After recent injury, fracture, or surgery, wait until the swelling and bruising heals substantially. (You can *Gua Sha* the surrounding areas while waiting until the site of the surgery or injury is healed.)

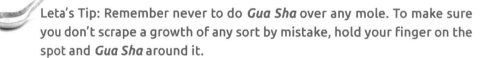

Leta's Tip: You can *Gua J* fairly soon after injury on muscle groups that feed into and out of the affected area to relax the area, while avoiding the actual injured area. After a day or two with a mild injury, you can do *Gua Sha* as long as there isn't any intense pain associated with the scraping. In this case, start very lightly just to get the *qi* moving and test the person's pain level.

- **Over moles, warts, boils, carbuncles, abrasions, ulcers, skin tags, hives, lesions, black heads, or blemishes.**

Leta's Tip: Remember never to do *Gua Sha* over any mole. To make sure you don't scrape a growth of any sort by mistake, hold your finger on the spot and *Gua Sha* around it.

- **Over varicose veins.** Avoid any veins that are visibly swollen or purple.
- **Over sunburned areas.** (Although *Gua Sha* can be useful on the scalp and the back of the neck as well as the upper back when you have heat exhaustion.)
- **Where there are open wounds.** Do not do *Gua Sha* on open wounds, ever.

- **Where there are rashes or inflamed skin.** Work around any rashes or inflamed skin to avoid causing the skin to break open.

Be cautious with the following people

- **Someone who is elderly or frail.** The elderly often have skin that is much thinner and more sensitive. In addition, if someone is very sick or frail, use very light pressure. Take more breaks; go more slowly.
- **Babies and children.** Lighter pressure. Always remember to tell parents to warn caregivers about markings.
- **Someone who is blood deficient or anemic.** People who are what we call "blood deficient" in Chinese Medicine may test positive for anemia or they may not technically be anemic, just close to anemic. If someone gets dizzy, lightheaded, or faint after receiving *Gua Sha*, they may be blood deficient. When the blood rises to the surface, there is less blood in their bodies, and they're already at a deficit. Have them rest and see a professional Chinese Medicine practitioner. The person may need to have *moxabustion* (a technique that nourishes the blood and helps those who are anemic) to balance their *Gua Sha* treatment.
- **Someone who has Fibromyalgia.** Fibromyalgia is a pain in the $#@% –literally! People with fibromyalgia sometimes report having a lot of pain *during and after* their initial *Gua Sha* treatment. (*Gua Sha* normally does not hurt after the session except for an occasional small amount of tenderness in the area for most people.) Fibromyalgia clients can sometimes be extremely sensitive and bruise easily. You can do a short session with very light pressure as a test. For those who experience tenderness and a lot of heat rising to the surface, they can apply *Zheng Gu Shui* or an arnica gel like Traumeel for the next 24 hours or so.

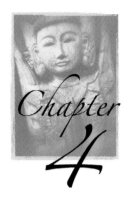

Chapter
4

THE GUA SHA 101'S

It's time to grab a spoon and get started! Okay, so how do you actually do *Gua Sha*? Here are my basic guidelines for starting out.

- Before beginning any session (even if it is just on yourself) turn off the room's air conditioner, or move out of the direct flow of the cold air. Because *Gua Sha* is used to release the effects of the Wind in the body, doing *Gua Sha* in the wind (fan or air conditioning included) doesn't make a lot of sense.

- Begin with applying oil to the area. I prefer organic coconut oil due to its consistency and its lasting a very long time. You can use a massage lotion, but often the spoon simply wipes it off the skin, necessitating that you reapply the lotion over and over again—not too much fun.

- Grip the spoon firmly. You can hold the spoon in two ways. (*See illustrations on opposite page.*)

1. With the top facing upward, place your thumb at the base of the handle. Now turn the top of the spoon toward the recipient's skin and rub the skin with the spoon's edge (the edge farthest from you as shown in the five pictures on page 28).

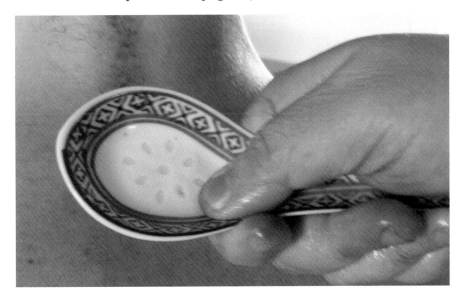

2. An alternative way to hold the spoon is upside-down with your thumb at the base of the handle.

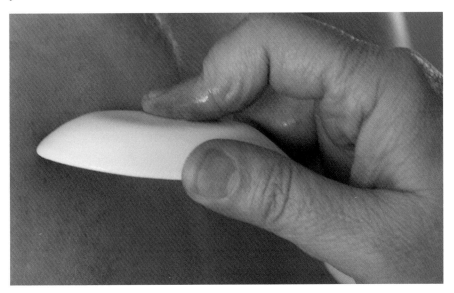

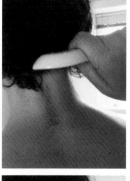

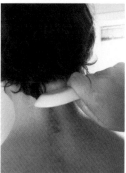

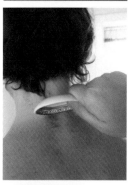

- Apply pressure in six-inch strokes or smaller, depending on the size of the area. You should *Gua Sha* for 30 to 60 seconds in an area to see if any *Sha* appears.

- Start with a light pressure for everyone. Ask the recipient how that feels. Does it feel kind of like massage? Or does it feel uncomfortable? Ticklish? Painful in any way? If they feel pain or discomfort, explain to them that you can do it more lightly, and then lessen the pressure so they can feel the difference. Ask if the lighter touch feels more comfortable. If they are ticklish, I find a bit harder pressure may prove better. If a lot of *Sha* is coming out in that area, assure them that it should begin to feel better soon if they want to continue.

- Mostly *Sha* will arise in the first 20 seconds. But some people are blood deficient. They've been told that they are anemic or you might notice that they have a very pale tongue. In this case, reduce the pressure you are applying. Be aware that bringing out the *Sha* might take quite a bit longer. Blood doesn't rise to the surface in blood deficient people as fast as it normally would. Sometimes when I see a tiny bit of *Sha*, I'll spend much longer on that area to make sure that I don't miss the emerging *Sha*.

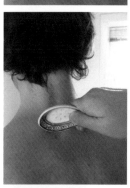

- In some cases, if a person is very tight and tense, the *Sha* won't come out right away due to the person tensing up. I encourage that individual to relax and to let the tension go or release. If the person can then relax, the *Sha* usually will come out quickly in a burst of redness.

Leta's Tip: Cramp alert! You almost *never Gua Sha* the whole body, just the areas that need attention. (It can be exhausting to the recipient to have too much work done in a single session.) Start with 15 minutes of *Gua Sha* and rest. You'll benefit too. Working up slowly will help your hands adjust to the work they are doing, and cramping will subside. Make sure you find a *Gua Sha* tool you like in order to avoid the over-cramping of your hand.

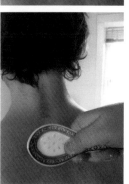

- When working on pain, make sure you start on a higher spot on the body. If the pain is anywhere on the arm or fingers for example, start on the back of the neck or the pecs on the front of the body, depending on which fingers or sides of the arms are affected. Learning the meridians of the arms and legs can be very helpful and is essential for the professional or frequent practitioner. For example, if a person feels numbness and tingling in their pinkies, that could be a sign that the Small Intestine meridian, which passes through the neck and the back of the shoulder blades, is tense, holding resistance, or blocked. You will often find a lot of *Sha* in the shoulder blades in this case. We will discuss the arm meridians in Chapter 5.

Practice, practice, practice, and rest!

Gua Sha can cause muscle strain in the practitioner, especially if you're a beginner. It takes a lot of forearm strength and can cause some pain in the wrist or fingers as well. As a beginner, start with short periods of *Gua Sha*. You'll usually want to use your dominant hand, but learning to do it with both hands can help when one hand is beginning to hurt. It takes some time to build up the muscle strength to do long sessions of *Gua Sha* (for example an entire back with a lot of *Sha*).

Whether on yourself or a recipient, you need to find positions that do not put strain on your wrists or shoulders. You will need to experiment in the beginning to find where you can best stand and how you should hold your arm.

When using the *Gua Sha* spoon, you want to employ a scooping motion, like a small arc. These repetitive strokes may cause pain in the wrist at first, so proceed slowly. Let your wrists and arms get used to this new motion. You don't want to simply rub the spoon on the skin. You want your arm, hand, and fingers to achieve a uniform stroke with an upward flicking motion at the end. Again, 30 to 45 degrees from the skin's surface is good. Visit: www.GuaShaBook.com to see videos of the flicking motion.

Leta's tip: Technically speaking, the energy that is being released by *Gua Sha* is toxic energy. It is extremely important to wash your hands *after Gua Sha* even if they look clean. The oils of the person's skin containing the toxins that are being released will mix into the oils you apply. So it's important to keep yourself and your tools clean afterwards.

What if fluid is released?

Gua Sha should never be done so hard as to cut the skin or cause the release of bodily fluids. However, if fluid is released from some bumps or pimples under the skin, quickly and gently wipe it away with a tissue and then wash your hands thoroughly. Clean the *Gua Sha* tool before proceeding (sterilization is best) or use a new tool. It's important to start with a sterilized utensil if you're using it in your healing practice. But even at home, cleanliness is always imperative, especially due to these occasional fluid eruptions.

After *Gua Sha-ing*

After performing a *Gua Sha* treatment, tell the recipient:

• Avoid extreme temperature changes for a short time afterward (no shower for at least 5 hours to allow your pores time to fully close).

• It might be prudent not to swim in cold water for the rest of that day.

• If it is windy and cold outside, ask the person to cover their skin to avoid repeated exposure.

• Take the rest of the day off. I always suggest that someone with an injury take it easy the rest of the day. If you're working on someone's arm, for example, and it feels completely better, it's still a good idea for them to rest it until the next day. If someone is fighting off a cold and feels much better, it's probably wise for them not to go to the gym that night. Suggest that they go home and get some rest instead.

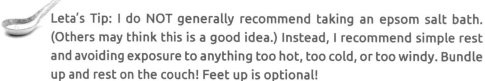

Leta's Tip: I do NOT generally recommend taking an epsom salt bath. (Others may think this is a good idea.) Instead, I recommend simple rest and avoiding exposure to anything too hot, too cold, or too windy. Bundle up and rest on the couch! Feet up is optional!

- Diet matters. If you are fighting off a cold, eat well (no fried or heavy dairy foods). Limit alcohol and avoid super cold foods like ice cream.

Reading the signs . . . following the *red path*

Gua Sha often has immediate results. If you have body pain, the pain may disappear. If it's a cold, you may immediately feel much relief. It usually depends on how far the cold has progressed.

Gua Sha also gives us a lot of information. For example, one man I worked on had forearm pain but couldn't remember doing anything to cause the pain. He was surprised when all of the *Sha* came out in his neck, shoulder, and upper arm. In other words, none of the *Sha* emerged at the site of the pain. However, after doing the session, he reported that the pain was completely gone! How'd that work? Well, this pain was being caused from something along the same meridian, just above the pain site, in this case, the forearm. Once the *Sha* was released, all the blood and *qi* started flowing again in the arm, and then the pain in the forearm disappeared!

Gua Sha is only skin deep

Gua Sha is a surface treatment. It works on the skin, muscles, and surface tendons. It's not meant to be done on a very deep level or with hard pressure. For areas that have chronic deep pain in the joints or that are deep below the surface (for example over the buttocks and hips), *Cupping* (a Chinese Medicine technique that applies suction cups to an area) can be a good follow-up to *Gua Sha*. Cupping is used to access deeper areas such as the buttocks and hips for pain where *Gua Sha* is less effective. Often this kind of deep pain comes from a chronic condition. One woman I worked with had experienced hip pain for 10 years. She felt some relief from *Gua Sha*, but after three applications of cupping, the pain disappeared completely. Some people apply cups and drag them across the skin (called "dragging cupping"), which is similar to the *Gua Sha* technique. Dragging cupping releases *Sha* through suction instead of scraping. I humorously like to call it "Dragon Cupping" since it can be intense!

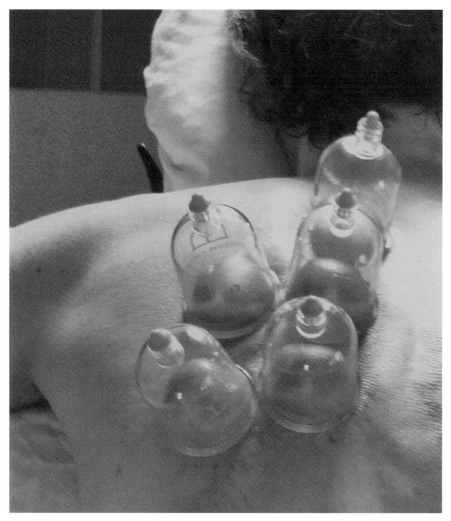

In general, *Gua Sha* releases toxins that are on the surface of the body, and cupping is for drawing out toxins that are closer to the bones and joints deep in the body.

Chapter 5

COLDS AND FEVER
AND FLU, OH MY!

Chinese Medicine is centered on the belief that every person is unique and what works to heal one person does not necessarily work for everyone. With this in mind, as a beginner, you need to be observant of someone you plan to work with and ask questions.

This chapter will help you take into consideration some of the many, many variables I've seen with different kinds of ailments and pain. These are not recipes but rather guidelines for specific conditions you may want to use *Gua Sha* for. As we've explained many times in this book, use your best judgment and seek medical advice in any case that involves a serious illness, communicable disease, high fever, or severe infection. *Gua Sha* is only meant to help someone in the following cases and should never be a substitute for medical attention. If you're not sure, ask a doctor or a Chinese Medicine practitioner.

Cold/flu/fevers/allergies

Colds that are caused by "Wind," can be easily nipped in the bud before they worsen. I follow these techniques in my practice:

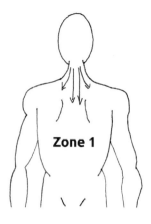

Zone 1

1. I start by *Gua Sha-ing* one of three zones (you can *Gua Sha* all of them if you don't know which one is best):

Zone 1 – The back of the neck is especially important for someone who is just getting a cold, at the first sign of symptoms. This phase of a cold is called a *"Wind Cold"* condition in Chinese Medicine.

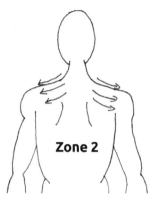

Zone 2

Zone 2 - The tops of shoulders (trapezius muscles) down to the middle of the back, including shoulder blades, is especially good for colds that have been around a while with a lot of phlegm. Often you may see a thick white or yellow coat on the recipient's tongue that looks like a sticky paste. This phase of a cold is called a *"Damp Heat"* condition in Chinese Medicine.

Zone 3 - The sides of the ribs and under the breasts is especially good for infections. This phase of a cold or type

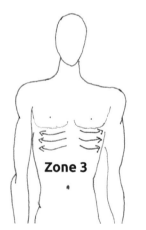

Zone 3

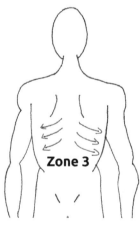

Zone 3

of illness is called a *"Wind Heat"* condition in Chinese Medicine. Sometimes nasty viruses, like the flu, last for a week or two and become *"Wind Heat"* conditions. Other conditions that are called *"Heat in the Blood"* in Chinese Medicine correspond to this zone. These include conditions such as Shingles, Poison Ivy Infections, Cellulitis, Staph, or other types of infections.

 Leta's Tip: While *Gua Sha* can be very helpful for *"Heat in the Blood"* types of infections, you must seek medical attention for such conditions. These can be life-threatening and need immediate medical care. In addition to standard Western medical treatments, *Gua Sha* can be performed by a professional Chinese Medicine practitioner. When in doubt, go to the doctor or emergency room.

2. After I do *Gua Sha*, I add specific acupressure points, especially *Jing-Well* points (see below).

Leta's Tip: A discussion of which acupressure points to use for specific cold symptoms would be such a large topic, it needs (and will get) its own book! Learn these **Jing-Well** points described below. They are always helpful for any **Gua Sha** session because they release energy to the exterior.

Nail them every time!

The *Jing-Well* points are all the points on the fingernails and toenails. They are useful for times when the *Gua Sha* release is extensive, and the person feels strange sensations coming out of their hands and feet. After *Gua Sha*, to be sure to get a better release of the Wind, you can work the nail points of the associated meridians. The nail points release any Wind that wasn't released through the skin during *Gua Sha*.

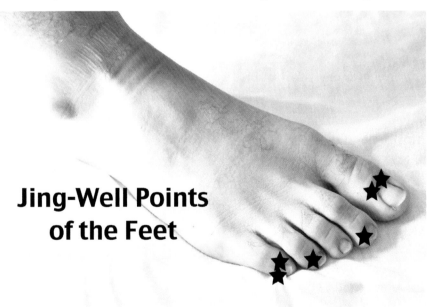

Jing-Well Points
of the Feet

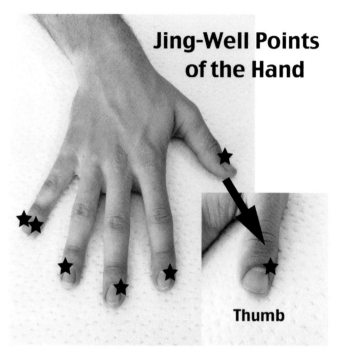

Jing-Well Points of the Hand

Thumb

Sometimes when you perform *Gua Sha*, the "Wind" gets stimulated and moves to other areas of the body instead of releasing. Sometimes people say the pain is traveling around their body when you do *Gua Sha*. In these cases, the Jing-Well points help release the Wind in the affected meridians.

To perform acupressure on a nail point, place your finger on the point. Now pump your finger up and down. While pulsating, focus on releasing the energy as you come up. Another technique is to lightly scrape the nail point (toward the tip of the finger). In ancient times this technique was called "chiseling" and was administered using a "needle" that was the shape of a chisel. Thankfully we have found a different way!

Coughs

In my experience, coughs are the hardest of all the cold symptoms to shift right away. However, I've found that *Gua Sha* is actually one of the best techniques to relieve coughing symptoms in my clients. I use the following approaches:

1.   I typically do *Gua Sha* on the back behind the lungs first. I do not add *Gua Sha* on the chest unless necessary. Many people with nasty coughs (that have been around for a while) are feeling quite weak, and *Gua Sha* on the front of the chest can be tiring.

2.   For severe coughs, I sometimes *Gua Sha* the front of the chest lightly. If the person is very weak, do not apply *Gua Sha*. For a strong

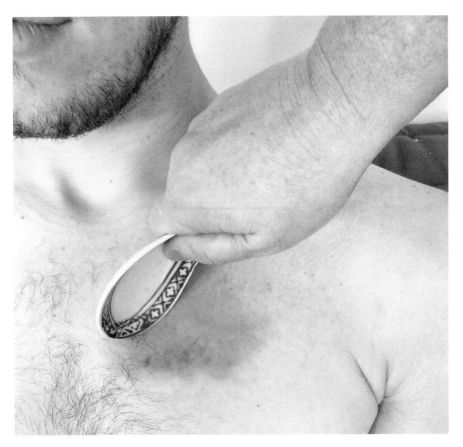

person with persistent chronic cough, I usually do a little *Gua Sha* on the front, and see if there's a lot of red. If so, *Gua Sha* the whole area. *Gua Sha* can also be used to reduce the severity of coughing fits.

Leta's Tip: For pneumonia, bronchitis, and walking pneumonia, seek medical attention. In addition to standard Western medical treatments, *Gua Sha* can be performed by a professional Chinese Medicine practitioner.

Heat exhaustion

Heat exhaustion can come from overexposure to the sun or heat without proper hydration. I never *Gua Sha* sunburns, but I do find *Gua Sha* on the scalp, back of the neck, and upper back helpful for relieving symptoms of heat exhaustion.

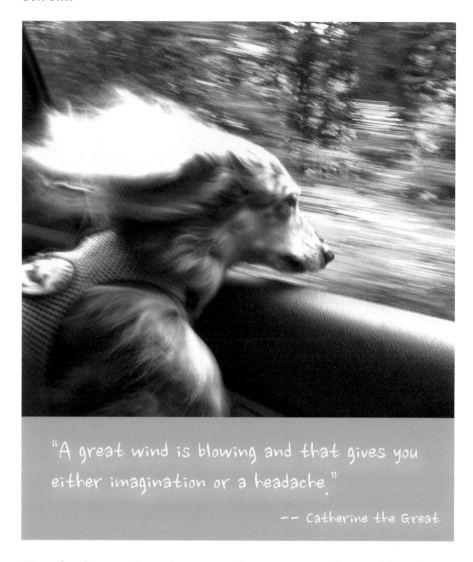

"A great wind is blowing and that gives you either imagination or a headache."

—— Catherine the Great

Headaches, migraines, and stress . . . three biggies!

There are many kinds of headaches and migraines. There are headaches in the back of the head, in the front of the head, or those on the side (usually one-sided). I do find *Gua Sha* particularly helpful for headaches in the back of the head and for some one-sided headaches.

For headaches in back of the head:

• I find if you apply *Gua Sha* to the back of the neck for headaches that start in the back of the head, many people find immediate relief. Remember to *Gua Sha* from the neck upward into the occiput (back of the skull). (*See illustration on p. 22.*)

For one-sided headaches:

•   Do the neck area mentioned above and **add** *Gua Sha* on the sides of the back of the neck.

Other headaches:

•   Do both areas of the neck mentioned above and **add** *Gua Sha* on the scalp.

•   With general headaches, I also add *Gua Sha* down the back, especially along both sides of the spine.

•   You can also *Gua Sha* across the tops of the shoulders, especially for one-sided headaches.

•   Add *Gua Sha* on any other areas of stress that the person reports or that you notice look tense.

Leta's Tip: When doing *Gua Sha* on the scalp, you might not be able to see the *Sha* beneath the hair, but light scraping on the scalp feels great and can immediately relieve the pain.

Working against the pain

To help heal pain, I always start higher on the body than where the person indicates the location of the pain to be. Here is a series of steps I work through with a client who is having pain.

1.   I find the meridian that runs through the area of pain. I follow the meridian pathway up. For example, for hand or wrist pain, I do *Gua Sha* on the neck, shoulder, and chest areas to see if any *Sha* appears there. Or for feet and legs, I start in the low back and sacrum areas.

2.   I *Gua Sha* the meridian lines down to the area of pain. For example, if the thumb hurts, I follow the Lung meridian from the pectoral muscles on the chest down to the wrist to see if red appears along that entire line.

3.   I check the nearby meridians. Often the meridian that runs through the painful location isn't the original source of the pain or other meridians were "recruited" to help with the pain and protect an injury.

Leta's Tip: For injuries, do not *Gua Sha* any contusions or swollen/hot areas. You can *Gua Sha* above and below such areas to increase the *qi* flow through the area. Wait until bruising or swelling is reduced before doing *Gua Sha* on the site of an injury. Such a treatment can be very helpful for chronic pain at the site of an old injury, after the healing process is further along.

4. For stubborn pains, I would suggest using *Gua Sha* in conjunction with *Sinew Channel* acupressure treatments, which release muscle groups through active resistance and acu-points. A Chinese Medicine practitioner trained in *Sinew Channel* treatments could help.

Leta's Tip: *Gua Sha* can help people who have pain from repetitive stress, such as musicians, athletes, or heavy computer users. It's important to explain that they need to go a little easier. A little more each day. Pain from repetitive stress comes when they first change something they're doing and expect new muscles to be as strong as the ones that have been built up over time. When they make changes to their routine, they have to act like a beginner and go a little easier. A little each day. Use *Gua Sha* to help with this process, but warn them that pain could come back intensely if they go gung-ho again.

Pain in the neck is, well, a pain in the neck!

When working with someone's neck, I do *Gua Sha* with clients sitting up since I can access their back, front, and the sides of their neck in this position.

Neck pain is typically either in the back or the side of the neck.

1. I ask the person where the pain is and start *Gua Sha* there.
2. After I complete the *Gua Sha* in all the red areas, I make sure to extend to the edge of the redness. (This might mean going quite far down the back, into the shoulder blades, or across the top of the shoulders.)

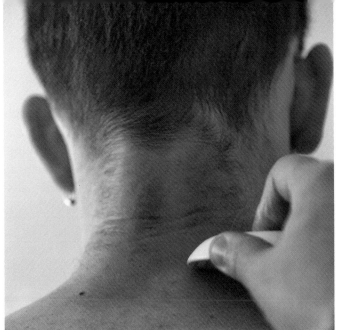
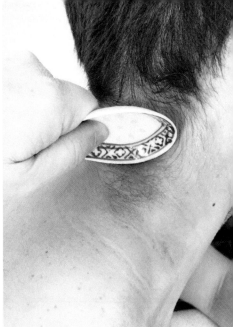

3.   I then ask clients to turn their necks and rotate their shoulders. Where do they still feel pain? Sometimes they will point to a completely different place.

4.   Wherever they point, I *Gua Sha* that spot to ensure I've gotten all the *Sha* out of it. Often someone might point to the top of an arm or shoulder when all neck pain is done. I then *Gua Sha* any area where they still feel pain.

5.   If pain persists, I do "moving" *Gua Sha*, which is doing *Gua Sha* while the person moves in a way that activates a painful muscle.

6.   To test what direction to move the neck, I put my hand on the area of pain and feel the aggravated muscle. I then ask the person to move the neck in various directions (up, down, side-to-side) to determine which motion utilizes that neck muscle.

7.   Once I determine the motion that best activates the muscles in the painful area, I ask the person to slowly, repeatedly, move that way while I perform *Gua Sha* on the area. For example, if pain is on the right side of the neck, I ask clients to rotate their head completely to the left. Now, while they slowly move the neck back to the right, I administer *Gua Sha* to the same spot. I then ask them to repeat the same motion while I *Gua Sha* the surrounding muscles (a wider area around that muscle).

This treatment usually takes care of whatever stubborn, remaining pain exists. The rule here is: Be patient with your patient.

The weight of the world can get heavy: Shoulder pain

I typically perform *Gua Sha* on the shoulders with the recipient sitting up so that I can access both the front and back sides of the body easily. Then I have the recipient lie down when I need to focus on the pectoral muscles (since it's a bit easier ergonomically to have them lie down for work on the front of the body).

1.   I start doing *Gua Sha* in the neck area and move down. I usually like to go over the mid-arm thoroughly, since the *deltoid* shoulder muscles attach to the *deltoid tuberosity* (a bony area in the *bicep* area of the arm).

2.   I often add *Gua Sha* under the armpit or under the back of the shoulder blade.

 Leta's Tip: To *Gua Sha* the *infraspinatus* muscle (under the shoulder blade), I ask clients to hold the opposite shoulder with their hand. This opens the shoulder blade to give access to the muscles underneath.

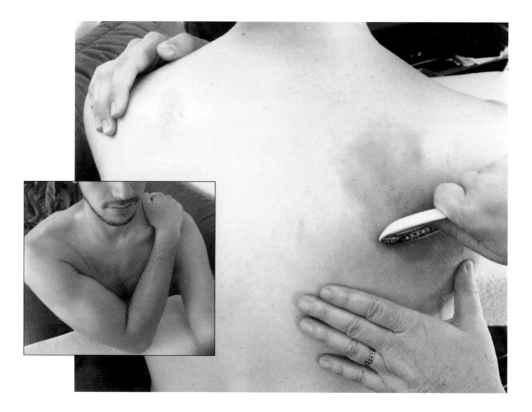

Carpal tunnel, carpal tunnel, carpal tunnel, carpal tunnel, carpal tunnel . . . (you get the idea)

Carpal Tunnel Syndrome is pain on the inside of your forearm caused by repetitive motion. I've found *Gua Sha* to be extremely helpful with carpal tunnel-like pain and symptoms.

1.   I usually start with the person sitting up to access the neck and shoulders. Once I descend to the arm, then I have the person lie down.

2.   I then evaluate which meridians are involved, based on the person's symptoms. The inside of the arm is made up of three meridians: Lung, Pericardium, and Heart:

• The Lung meridian extends from your collar bone to your thumb.

• The Pericardium meridian extends from your Pectoral muscles (just above the breast) to your middle finger.

• The Heart meridian extends from your armpit to your pinkie (inner nail corner).

3.   I then ask recipients if they have any numbness, tingling, or pain in any finger. This often indicates which meridian to focus on first.

4.   After determining which meridians are involved, I start at the top (collarbone, pectorals, or armpit area) and work my way down. You can check all three meridians to be sure.

5.   While I occasionally get *Sha* in the forearm, typically more *Sha* will come out in the Pectoral muscles or the upper arm area.

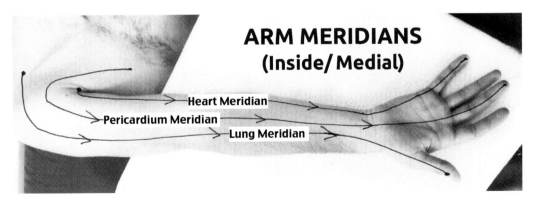

**ARM MERIDIANS
(Inside/Medial)**

Heart Meridian
Pericardium Meridian
Lung Meridian

Pain on the top of the forearm

Some people think they have carpal tunnel, but all their pain is on the outside/top of their forearm. It can be confusing. To work on this area, I use similar techniques as described above in the carpal tunnel section.

1. To access the neck and shoulders, I start with the person sitting up. Then as I move downward working on the arm, I have the person lie down to make access to the arm even easier.

2. I then evaluate which meridians are involved based on the

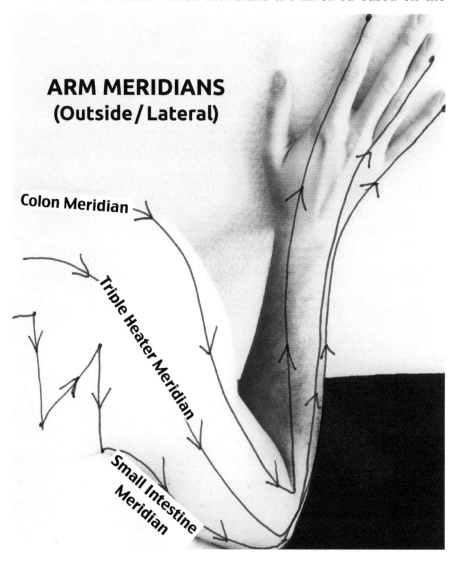

ARM MERIDIANS
(Outside / Lateral)

Colon Meridian

Triple Heater Meridian

Small Intestine Meridian

person's symptoms. The top of your forearm is made up of the following meridians:

- The Colon meridian extends from the front of the neck, over the middle of the shoulder, through the crook of the elbow to the forefinger.
- The Triple Heater (*San Jiao*) meridian extends from the side of the neck over the top/back of the shoulder, to the funny bone, and finally to the ring finger.
- The Small Intestine meridian travels from the side of the neck to the back of the shoulder blade, to the back of the armpit, through the back of the elbow, and finally to the pinky (outer pinky nail corner).

3. I then ask clients if they have any numbness, tingling, or pain in any finger. These sensations are often indicators of which meridian to focus on first.

4. Once I determine which meridians are involved in the pain, I start at the top (the neck, shoulder, or back of shoulder) and work my way down. You can check all three meridians to be sure.

5. While I'll occasionally get *Sha* in the forearm, typically more *Sha* will come out in the neck, top of the shoulder, or shoulder blade.

Leta's Tip: For hand or finger pain, proceed as you would with arm pain, paying special attention to which fingers hurt. You can *Gua Sha* the wrist and hand as well, even the fingers themselves!

Leta's Tip: Numbness and tingling can be greatly helped with *Gua Sha*. Often people experience numbness and tingling that wakes them up at night. The source is often found in the Small Intestine or Triple Heater meridians, but can be any of the arm meridians.

The big, bad, nasty back pains

I tend to think of back pain as three types: upper, middle, and lower back pain.

- **Upper back pain**

I begin at the neck and work the top of the shoulders and the upper back entirely. I add the shoulder blades if a lot of *Sha* appears there.

- **Mid-back pain**

I start at the neck, go down the sides of the spine, and focus on the middle back, into the ribs. (See if the *Sha* wraps around to the sides of the ribs, wrapping around to the front of the body . . . follow the redness.)

- **Lower back pain**

This can be more mysterious and is a bit more advanced. Often pain is at the center of the back, near the spine or on the sacrum, but I always make sure to extend the *Gua Sha* out to the sides of the low back. Often I get much more *Sha* at the sides than in the

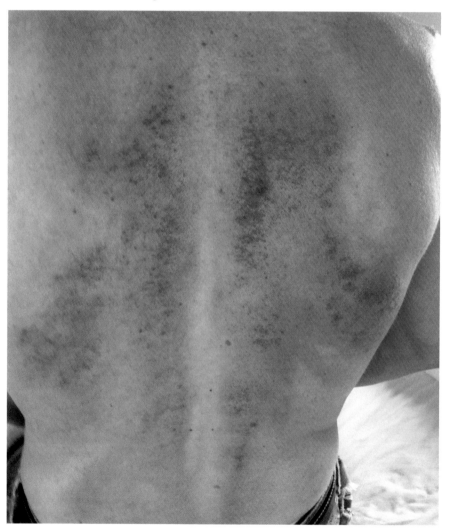

center, and this seems to be key to releasing the pain in the middle. To do the sacral area, I have them lie down on their belly. For low back pain, I also include the buttocks, especially the center of each cheek where the Piriformis muscle is located. I also find it necessary to use more pressure in this fleshier area. Don't be afraid. I often repeatedly check with the recipient to make sure it's not painful from the additional pressure.

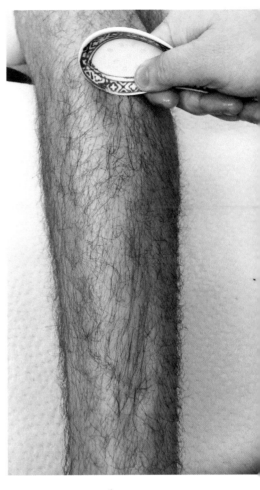

Leg/knee/foot pain

Just like arm pain, you need to be aware of where the pain is coming from when working on the legs and lower extremities. The meridians of the back of the leg go up into the sacrum and hips. The meridians of the front of the leg go up into the groin area. Here are some tips:

- **Shin Splints** often just need *Gua Sha* on the site of the pain (front of the lower leg, on the top of the *tibia*, and to the outer (lateral) side of the *tibia* into the *fibula* area (outside of the leg).

- **Sciatica**–Sciatica pain can have various causes. For example, you need to know what kind of sciatica the person is experiencing. There are two types:

  - Bladder sciatica–shoots down the back of the legs
  - Gall Bladder sciatica–shoots down the sides of the legs

I find that most sciatica pain needs *Gua Sha* on the low back, hip, and sacral area. For Bladder channel pain, I work the sacrum. For Gall Bladder pain, I work the hip area and the *greater trochanter* (bony area below the hip). Also for Gall Bladder sciatica, I lightly *Gua Sha* the *Iliotibial* (IT) Bands. This area can be very painful on just about everyone, so proceed lightly and ask about your pressure levels. Other acupressure techniques might be very useful for stubborn sciatica.

Leta's Tip: Sciatica can have several causes, including possible trouble with your spine. For painful, persistent sciatica, seek a medical evaluation and then talk to a Chinese Medicine practitioner.

- **Plantar Fasciitis** or foot pain has various causes. For this reason, it's more complex to work out what plan of action to take. I generally work on a number of different areas until I get results.
  - I usually start by doing *Gua Sha* on the back of the calf and the inside of the calf (these are the Bladder and Kidney channels, respectively).
  - I sometimes *Gua Sha* the bottom of the foot as well, very lightly since it can be quite painful for people with plantar fasciitis.

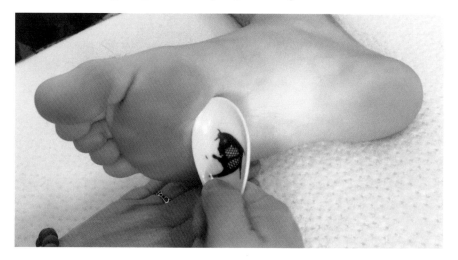

  - I also check to see if there's any *Sha* in the low back and sacral areas.
  - I also combine *Gua Sha* with other acupressure techniques in stubborn cases.

Leta's Tip: It's important that the person get a medical evaluation to ensure there isn't a fracture or other problem in the foot that could require surgery. It's not very common, but I always recommend having it checked to avoid months of needless pain. Follow up with a Chinese Medicine practitioner.

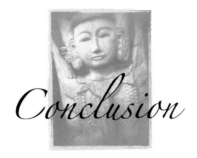

Conclusion

CLOSING THOUGHTS

We're thrilled to share what we've learned about *Gua Sha* with you. As an ancient healing art, we believe it's a safe and effective tool for healing. We are also extremely fortunate to have modern medicine and technology at our disposal. Just because modern medicine is so good at saving lives and diagnosing serious illness does not mean we need to ignore centuries of medicine based on Chinese Medicine's simple goal of living long, healthy lives through "prevention and attention" to general health. One of our most important goals in writing this book (and teaching our classes) is to make simple, safe, and effective ancient healing techniques accessible to everyone, regardless of class, education, or financial status in life. *Gua Sha* levels the playing field (or in this case—the healing field) because anyone can do it. It is for anyone and everyone.

As always, use common sense in your own health or your healing practice. Modern medicine has many tools that are extremely useful for most serious medical conditions. We do encourage working with your doctor and learning more about alternative medicine therapies that might be useful for your particular condition (or are complementary to your healing practice if you are a practitioner).

Incorporating *Gua Sha* into your life

If you become an avid *Gua Sha*-er like we are, you may want to become a spoon-carrying citizen. Slip one into the pocket of your purse or briefcase, the glove box of your car, or your bedside table's drawer. When you need a spoon, you want it right away. Here's why:

1. **Catch colds BEFORE they start** – At the first throat tickle or sniffle, take out your spoon and immediately *Gua Sha* the back of your neck.

2. **If you overdo it at home** – A little too much yard work all day Sunday? Get your spoon out. Pulled a muscle playing soccer with the kids? Time to scrape away. Catch these minor pains before they become big pain.

3. **A little over-zealous working out** – The spoon is the athlete and weekend warrior's best friend. If you're always pushing yourself to do new and interesting activities, that means using new muscles that could complain for days afterwards. Use your spoon accordingly to be able to keep on going and going!

Adding a Spoonful of Medicine

If you have a healing or bodywork practice and are considering adding *Gua Sha* to your list of healing modalities, check the bylaws in your area. If you are currently a licensed practitioner, make sure *Gua Sha* falls into the scope of your practice.

• If you have a client who temporarily feels better after your treatments/sessions but the pain returns a day or two afterwards, *Gua Sha* may be very helpful. You could add this modality to your practice (if the law permits) or refer your client to a Chinese Medicine practitioner for *Gua Sha*.

• *Gua Sha* can be done for 5-10 minutes at the beginning of your session to relieve pain but also to assess the source of the pain.

Remember, the spoon does not lie! Wherever the redness appears is the area to focus on with your other work.

• The number one question I get from other practitioners who want to add *Gua Sha* to their practice is: "How do I introduce this to my existing clients?" My answer is always, "Be confident, enthusiastic, and explain the benefits of *Gua Sha* in a positive way."

The best thing about *Gua Sha* is you can just get your spoon and start spooning where it hurts. We hope this book will give you a more thorough understanding of what *Gua Sha* has to offer. If you want to continue with *Gua Sha*, this book can provide the information you need to become a more skilled practitioner. By understanding some general Chinese Medicine concepts, some meridians of the body, and a few essential acupressure concepts, you will be on your way!

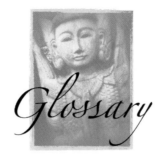

Glossary

The following are definitions of some terms we've used throughout the book.

Cupping - A Chinese Medicine technique that uses cups to apply suction to specific areas of the body to release deeper muscles and ligaments as well as stuck energy and blood in the joints.

Gua - The actual scraping technique.

Gua Sha - A healing technique that uses a tool to apply friction to the skin in order to release pain and stuck energy.

Jing-Well Points - The Acupressure points located on the nails of the fingers and toes that release Wind to the surface.

Moxa (Moxabustion) - A Chinese Medicine technique that is used to apply heat to acu-points or areas of the body. The practitioner lights the herb *artemisia vulgaris*, or mugwort, rolled into cones on specific points. Or the practitioner uses a moxa stick (moxa rolled into a long stick) to heat a larger area for pain relief. Moxa promotes blood and *qi* circulation and is very helpful for chronic pain.

Petechiae - The small red dots that emerge when doing *Gua Sha*. Also called *Sha*.

Sha - The red color that emerges from doing *Gua Sha* (or technically speaking, the energy that's released when the red colored areas appear).

Sinew Releases - A Chinese Medicine technique to release pain along the Sinew Meridians. The Sinew Meridians are a different set of meridians than the primary meridians that are used in most Chinese Medicine treatments. The Sinew Meridians are wide bands that correspond to many muscle groups. Sinew Meridian treatments involve the practitioner providing resistance so the recipient can activate the painful muscle while moving it, followed by acupressure techniques that release Wind.

Spooning and/or Scraping - our nicknames for *Gua Sha*.

Wind - An ancient metaphor for the type of energy that is released when doing *Gua Sha*.

Zones - There are three zones where *Gua Sha* can be applied to release Wind from the body: The back of the neck, the upper and mid-back, and the ribs.

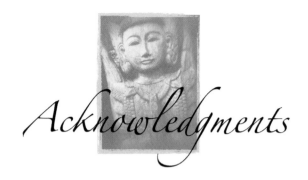

Acknowledgments

IN APPRECIATION

We are grateful to all who helped make this book come to life. Our heart-felt thanks go to Dr. Steve Herman, Jennifer Abbingsole, Debbie Tricarico, and Mia Craven, our tireless editors, who with great aplomb met our accelerated need to get this book published and in the hands of people around the world. Our gratitude to Michael Nelson for his wonderful work with the technical layout for our books. Also, to all who attended our *Gua Sha* workshop this year, asking astute questions and prompting us to write useful answers. Thank you, thank you, thank you. Together we are changing the world one spoon at a time (and laughing along the way really helps)!

Leta: I am so grateful for my teacher Jeffrey Yuen for so freely sharing his knowledge of *Gua Sha* and its many healing benefits.

Jaye: No recognition of gratitude could be complete without the acknowledgement of the big three in life: the Spark, the Rock, and the little Bark. I am so grateful to have everyone that I have in my life. Thank you!

ABOUT THE AUTHORS

LETA HERMAN is an author, Five Elements and Chinese Medicine teacher, nationally certified acupressure practitioner, and co-author of *The Energy of Love* (Llewellyn 2014) and *Connecting Your Circle* (*Born Perfect Ink* 2014). A Smith College graduate and former nationally syndicated journalist, Leta has immersed herself in the philosophies of Daoism, Alchemical Healing, and Chinese Medicine, as well as many other healing modalities. Leta has devoted the past fifteen years to learning everything possible about the Five Elements. In other aspects of life, Leta is also a world explorer who speaks multiple languages, loves life, her family, and can never resist a challenging game of Boggle.

JAYE McELROY is an author, photographer, business entrepreneur and co-author of *The Energy of Love* (Llewellyn 2014) and *Connecting your Circle* (*Born Perfect Ink* 2014). She considers herself a humble student of life, love, art, her most amazing dog Dax, and of course *Gua Sha* and the Five Elements. It has recently been discovered that one of her secret wishes in life is to travel through time and space in the Tardis with the Doctor. Who?

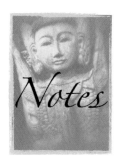

Notes

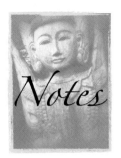

Notes

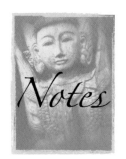

Notes

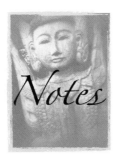

Notes

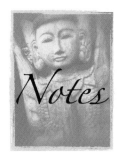

Notes

Please sign up for our newsletter and upcoming information on the soon to be released Five Element Series *"So You think you are..."* at:

www.ConnectingYourCircle.com
or
www.BornPerfectInk.com

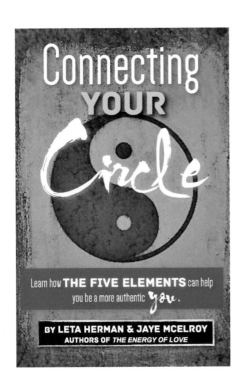

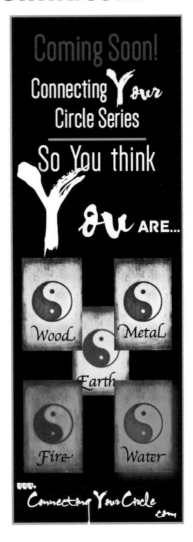

Available today at:
www.ConnectingYourCircle.com
or on www.Amazon.com

Also by Leta & Jaye...

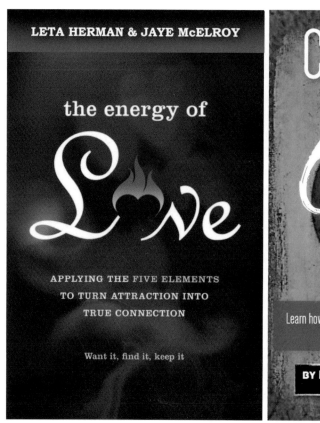

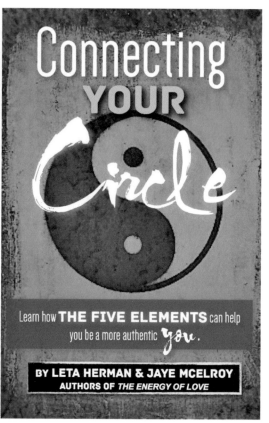

Available in bookstores & online today!

www.EnergyofLoveBook.com

www.ConnectingYourCircle.com

For any contact information, please visit:

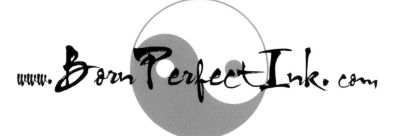

www.BornPerfectInk.com

CPSIA information can be obtained at www.ICGtesting.com
Printed in the USA
LVIW01n1717210515
439402LV00003B/20